CONTENTS

OUR BABY

Our Love

OUR LOSS

OUR BABY

Our Love

OUR LOSS

KATHI EVANS, BSN, RNC

Our Baby, Our Love, Our Loss

Published by Wheatmark™
610 East Delano Street, Suite 104, Tucson, Arizona 85705 U.S.A.
www.wheatmark.com
ISBN: 978-1-58736-730-4
LCCN: 2006939858

Unless otherwise indicated, Bible quotations are taken from the New King James Version of the Bible. Copyright © 1985 by Thomas Nelson, Inc.

Passages from New International Version: Copyright © 2002 Zondervan.

Artwork by Connie Beecher
at Butterfly Studios.
Contact at newcreationart@aol.com
Edited by Kathy Furlong.

ACKNOWLEDGMENTS

A s I BEGAN to think about the people I should express gratitude to for the impact they've had on my life since Peanut's birth and therefore on this book, I realized how incredibly God has blessed me with "encouragers," or "balcony people," as Joyce Landorf Heatherly puts it in her book *Balcony People.* These are the people who stand on the balcony of your life, looking down, cheering you on.

Pastors, my spiritual family, family members, friends, co-workers: these are the precious ones who have and continue to influence my life and whom I pray will see my gratitude to them by the way I love and encourage them in return. May God allow me to bless you in the same measure that He has used you to bless me!

I also want to "praise God from whom *all* blessings flow." Abba, Daddy, you have proved

Your love, faithfulness, long-suffering, and grace to me – to *me*! – over and over again. I love and thank you; help me to love and thank you more.

Mark, my love, the only way I could ever thank you for who you are to me and how God has used you in my life is to love, support and encourage you in like manner. In particular, thank you for the accountability and sometimes much-needed admonishments you've given me. Your heart's desire has always been to keep me on track, and you have!

Jason, I am so grateful for the lessons that God has taught me through you. You are so willing to encourage me, yet I know that the encouragement is never sugar-coated but is based on what you truly believe – whether I like it or not! Everyone needs people like that in their lives. You are one of God's blessings to me and I love you bunches!

Diana, thank you for loving me so much more than I deserve. You encourage me more than you'll ever know here on earth.

Bob, like David, I believe that you are a "man after God's own heart." That is only one of the reasons why I continually thank God for uniting our hearts. Your willingness to and regular practice of doing honest self-evaluation inspires and humbles me.

Jim and Mickie, I so appreciate your willingness to both love me and be honest with me. It occurs to me that God knows I need an extra dose of people who love me in spite of myself. Thank you for always being there.

Connie Beecher, you are another one of God's blessing to me. You have a heart that loves to love. Thank you for showering me with it. I am honored that you call me sister. Thank you, also, for so generously sharing your talent with me. You have a God-given heart of an artist and there is no doubt that I am a better artist and person for it.

Kathy Furlong, as the reality of this book started to come to fruition God brought some uniquely special people beside me. You are without doubt on that list! Thank you for sacrificially sharing the talent God has given you. When God provides the editor how can a person go wrong?

To each person in this "great cloud of witnesses" both named and unnamed, thank you for giving of yourselves to me so freely. I love you all with an eternal love.

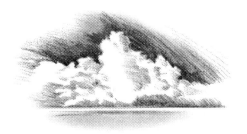

*Therefore we also, since we are surrounded
by so great a cloud of witnesses,
let us lay aside every weight, and the
sin which so easily ensnares us,
and let us run with endurance the
race that is set before us.*

Hebrews 12: 1

*This book is dedicated to every
precious little "Peanut"
and those who love them,
And to two of the best gifts
God has ever given me:
Mark and Jason.*

FOREWORD

Within 24 hours of delivering my second son at the beginning of the 16th week of pregnancy, much too early for him to live outside of the uterus, I began asking, "Why did I lose my baby boy?" I did not ask why in the sense of "why me?", you see I've known for a long time that there is nothing so special about me that I should be spared the hardships that are common to all of humanity. Rather, I asked, "What is the purpose for this loss? What does God want me to learn? How can I help others because of having suffered this tragedy?" Although the most important question I asked, at least to me, was, "Is there any way I can make sense of the most senseless thing I can imagine, the loss of a baby?"

Many years have come and gone since that July 24th, and during that time those questions have been answered in many different ways. As a registered nurse on a Labor and Delivery unit that averages around 200 deliveries per month, I've often had the opportunity to share my experience with couples who face the same kind of loss. It's gratifying to be able to say, "I know how you feel" and know that the parents can be assured that is true. While no one wants this type of education, with pain comes learning!

There have been times that I've met with fathers who have just lost a child, to share with them some of the things my husband, Mark, did for me that made our trial just a little easier. Those fathers often tell me that during the process of labor they feel helpless. They can't take the pain away, they are powerless to speed the process, and generally they feel inadequate in their role as "protector." With the birth of the baby all that changes, unless the baby is dead or soon will die. For those fathers, the pain of their loss compounds the feelings of helplessness and powerlessness. Mark showed me through our loss that, while the pain that comes with losing a baby is inevitable, there are things a father can do to help diminish those feelings of helplessness.

Being able to help a friend or family member through such a horrific loss just a bit more smoothly is yet another way God has shown me that our experience can have a positive impact. Have these situations made sense of the loss of my baby? Was his death worth the advantages I gained or the aid and advice I am able to give others? Without a doubt, *no*! I never would have chosen this path, but then it is not up to me to choose. The thing that I have gained is the knowledge that my child has made and continues to make a difference in this world. There is an incredible peace that comes to any parent who knows that to be true.

As the years passed and I "settled" into the role I felt God had chosen for me in relationship to the loss of our son, I began to feel somewhat comfortable doing this task to which I had been called. Then, suddenly, in a literal "blink of an eye", the thought came to me, "You should write a book." Of course, this thought was immediately dismissed! "Authors write books, philosophers write books, poets, scholars, and even cooks write books! But a mother who has lost one of her babies - she definitely is not on that list! That's especially true when that mother is me!" But the thought would not be persuaded to go away. I found that slowly, hesitantly, and very humbly I began to whisper in the deepest part of my heart where only God and I can hear, "With God's help maybe I can."

Even as you read the following chapters it is my desire that you know that I do not feel equal to this task. However, I've been blessed with some motivating factors: a deep and eternal love for my dear baby boy; the undying support of my husband and my oldest son, Jason; a burning desire to follow God's will for my life, *no matter what*; and a calling to do what I can to help moms and dads who are suffering through a similar loss, as well as their families, friends, doctors and nurses.

Not even one word of this book had been written when God "hit me on the head" with the title. Since then, however, it has become obvious that God and I had a small breakdown in our communications. (I wonder whose fault that was!) The title I originally had in mind for this book was, *My Baby, My Love, My Loss*. It was only after writing several of the chapters that I realized that it was an incredibly selfish and self-righteous title. This was certainly not only *my* baby. I definitely was not the only one who loved this baby. But mostly, how could I even imply that the burden of this loss was mine alone? The fact of the matter is, if I met this challenge with any graciousness or maturity, it is largely due to the measureless love, support and encouragement I received from my husband, in spite of the pain he himself was battling.

There was another reason that I needed to change the title. I dearly want to communicate to the reader that I am primarily addressing couples who have suffered the loss of a baby. While there are some aspects of this book that could prove helpful to single mothers going through this trial, I've based most of my feelings, observations and suggestions on our personal experience and the experiences of the couples I've been honored to provide nursing care for while they faced their loss. There are many issues and problems that a single mother endures that I have little or no experience with; therefore I would be out of line to try to offer advice to those women. If any of what I have to offer helps or encourages any single mothers, I give all the glory to God who does all things well.

While my initial intention was to help families who are trying to make sense of the loss they are feeling, God has brought to my attention there are other couples who might find help and encouragement in these pages: parents who have just learned that they have a special needs child. Both personally and professionally I've been given the privilege to walk down this challenging road with many people. In the process I've learned that when a family discovers that their precious baby will have special needs throughout life, they find themselves grieving the loss their "normal" child. Unfortunately, along with this grief often comes intense guilt. After all, in most ways their baby is physical healthy and alive.

If you find yourself on this journey, know that your feelings are normal, and I would even go as far as to say healthy. Allow yourself to grieve even as you rejoice over and love your baby. What an incredible paradox this season of your life has become! I pray that some of the suggestions I give in the last chapter will prove useful in resolving the dilemma you are facing a little more gracefully. I believe with all my heart that you will be a more loving and accepting parent in the future if you give yourself permission to grieve today.

So, does all of this answer the question, "Why?" Perhaps, although it is my belief that I will continue to ask and God will continue to answer that question for the rest of my life. There are probably answers to that question that I will never discover during this life. There is, however, comfort in knowing that God knows those answers and will withhold and reveal them as it is good and profitable for me. For God tells us, "The secret things belong to the Lord our God."(Deuteronomy 29:29) He also says, "Call to Me, and I will answer you, and show you great and mighty things, which you do not know." (Jeremiah 33:3) It is my deepest prayer that as you read the words before you, they will in some small way help you look to God to find the answers He has to this most important question.

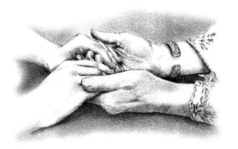

Do not let any unwholesome talk
come out of your mouths,
but only what is helpful for building
others up according to their needs,
that it may benefit those who listen.

Ephesians 4: 29 (NIV)

(Emphasis mine)

ONE

Our Story

DURING THE FIRST twelve weeks of pregnancy with my first son, Jason, I had a lot of trouble with bleeding and spent most of that time on bed rest, only getting up to go to the bathroom. At one point I even took sponge baths in bed and had my husband, Mark, washed my hair while I hung my head over the side of the bed; not an easy task in a water bed! At no point during this time, even with all the bleeding, did I have any pain, and this proved to be one of the greatest sources of hope for Mark and me. Then around the 12th week of the pregnancy the bleeding slowed down and by the 15th week I was able to return to work full time as a registered nurse on the Labor and Delivery unit in a large inner city hospital. In fact, I had to call in sick the day I went into labor, right on my due date!

In light of this, I was somewhat cautious when I started bleeding with my next pregnancy, but I wasn't nearly as frightened as I was the first time around. As with Jason, there was no pain with this bleeding either. I needed to be on bed rest, but not nearly as long. Each ultrasound showed everything to be normal. It was just a matter of waiting it out until the 12th week. I knew if I could make it that far that I would have it made.

We had planned a special week at a resort in the Pocono Mountains the week of Jason's fifth birthday in mid-July and were really hoping that my condition would be stable enough for us to go. Of course, we were prepared to cancel if necessary. Even though he would be disappointed, we knew that because Jason was so easy-going it wouldn't be a big problem, and we would make it up to him later. However, we were very hopeful about our plans because I would be the middle of my 14th week.

Several weeks before our vacation Jason began to refer to the baby as "her." This surprised us because we assumed that he would rather have a brother. But it also concerned us a little – we didn't want Jason to think of the baby as a particular gender and possibly be disappointed when the baby arrived. So, one night we had a family meeting and decided that we should give the baby a name that was neither male nor female that we could use until its arrival. After some discussion, we decided that since the baby was so tiny we would call it "Peanut." From that moment until he was born the "name" Peanut was spoken very often in the Evans' house.

I had been working part time since I returned to work after having Jason. So when the 12th week of my pregnancy came and the bleeding stopped, going back to work was a breeze, and we were reassured that everything was going to be all right. We began to get excited about our upcoming vacation and life getting back to normal. I even allowed myself to begin to wonder what life would be like with two children in the house!

Our vacation could not have been better! We had beautiful weather, the food at the resort was wonderful and our hearts practically burst with love for Jason, as he was so genuinely appreciative of every little thing we did for him. This was one of those special family times that will bring a smile to our faces when we sit on the porch in our rocking chairs and think about it in our retirement!

There was, however, one moment of concern during this otherwise perfect getaway. Just before we left for the resort, I had blood drawn one last time to measure the amount of progesterone in my body. One of the things that can cause bleeding and threaten a pregnancy in the first trimester is a low progesterone level. In a healthy pregnancy, the placenta begins to produce its own progesterone around the 12th week; until then, the hormone comes from the mother's body. Because of the bleeding I'd had, my doctors knew that I was not producing enough progesterone so hormone supplementation was prescribed and my levels were followed with repeated blood tests. In the middle of the week, I called the doctor to get the result of the blood test, anticipating that I would be able to stop taking the supplemental progesterone.

However, the news from the doctor was not good. We were hoping that the level had gone up although it wouldn't have been awful if it had stayed the same. But the progesterone level had gone down and I had to increase the dose I was taking. I also needed to see the doctor as soon as possible after we returned home.

Even so, we were encouraged by the fact that I felt fine and had no symptoms, not even the slightest bit of bleeding or pain. Yet we had a feeling of uneasiness that was difficult to shake. The remainder of our time together at the resort, although guarded, was just as delightful as before the phone call and we returned home without further complications.

We arrived home on Friday and I was scheduled to work night shift, 11:00p.m. to 7:00a.m. that weekend. I also had an appointment to see my obstetrician first thing Monday morning. We unpacked, Mark did a few loads of laundry, and we relaxed and enjoyed being home again.

The Saturday night shift proved to be uneventful until around 1:00 a.m. when I suddenly felt something that concerned me and went into the bathroom to assure myself that it was just my imagination. But there was nothing reassuring about what I saw: I had begun to bleed again, lightly and painlessly, but I knew that even this spotting was not good. Several thoughts reeled through my mind: "This isn't supposed to happen. I'm 15 weeks pregnant. The bleeding had stopped by this time with Jason."

I informed the charge nurse of what was happening and that I was calling my doctor. He, of course, instructed me to go home immediately on strict bed rest. After calling Mark, I very nervously did exactly what I was told.

After a few hours sleep, I awoke to discover that the bleeding had subsided and I had only a small amount of brownish discharge, a sign that there was no new bleeding. The doctor, Mark, and I felt somewhat relieved and we decided that I would remain on bed rest until my appointment the next morning. What happened next began one of the most horrible weeks of my life and put me on an emotional roller coaster like I had never before experienced.

About four o'clock in the afternoon I went into the bathroom. When I sat down on the toilet, blood began to pour out of me as if it were urine. I could not control it. I called for Mark to get me a towel. He then took Jason next door to his godparents and called the doctor's answering service to inform them that we were going to the hospital. Even though we live just blocks away and I put on a fresh pad held in place by a clean towel before leaving, both were saturated by the time we arrived at the hospital. I was trying to keep my hopes up by reminding myself that at least there was no pain.

Shortly after I arrived on the maternity floor and changed into the hospital gown, the bleeding pretty much stopped. The first thing to be done was to see whether or not Peanut survived this incredible episode. It was inconceivable to me that he could still be alive. Yet, there it was, that wonderful heartbeat as strong and steady as could be. I thought, "Peanut, my love, you must have an intense will to live!" Next came blood tests, IVs and an ultrasound. My iron level was a little low, which was to be expected, but the preliminary ultrasound showed nothing unusual. A more in-depth ultrasound was scheduled for Monday morning; until then I was on *complete* bed rest. I couldn't even eat, as it might become necessary for me to go to the operating room at any moment.

The ultrasound on Monday morning showed that a small corner of my placenta had pulled away from the wall of my uterus. This is called an abruption. Not knowing why this had happened was unsettling, but the abruption was small enough that it could heal over and I could still carry Peanut to term. However, it was also possible that it could happen again. Therefore, it was necessary for me to stay in the hospital a few days for observation and bed rest. At least I could eat and get up to go into the bathroom. With God's help, I thought, Peanut and I could do this.

However, it did happen again. In fact, every other day for the next four days I had a similar episode of bleeding. With each episode, it was as though God was gently whispering in my ear, "Kathi, I'm taking Peanut back, but I will let you have these last few days with him." As much as a mother possibly could, I enjoyed this time with Peanut. While Mark was with me as much as possible, Jason needed his attention also, perhaps more than I did. So I spent many hours alone in that bed.

Now, I was blessed that I had begun to feel Peanut move very early in the pregnancy. So, during those hours alone, I would put my hand over the place where Peanut was moving and I would gently push on it. Within a few seconds I would feel a little push back. It was as though Peanut was saying to me, "I feel you, Mommy, and I love you." In my heart I would answer back each time, "I love you too, Peanut." It was our prenatal game of "peek-a-boo!"

This would continue for several minutes at a time and then we would both rest until I felt Peanut's next tug at me saying, "I want to play!"

This was an intensely special time to me and I still smile at the thought of it. While I would not allow my head to think it, my heart knew that this was the closest I would come to getting a kiss from my sweet little Peanut. I didn't tell anyone about this for a long time for fear they'd think I was crazy. But I've come to realize that when something is that special to you, it doesn't matter what others think.

On Friday, July 24th, I received many warnings from those close to me that I should probably prepare myself for the inevitable. With each episode of bleeding the odds for Peanut's survival decreased. I knew this, but Peanut's life was in God's hands and I wasn't about to assume that He was going to take Peanut – after all, He is a God of miracles!

Around 4:00 p.m. my spirits were lifted by a visit from Mark and Jason. It was so refreshing to have Jason's youthful optimism and energy in the room. About the time they arrived I began to feel some gas pains, something that, unfortunately, has been a part of my genetic make-up since I was a little girl. The discomfort was annoying, but I ignored it and focused on my little blonde "ball of energy" running around the room, getting things for Mommy and occasionally giving me a pretend "pregestin" shot, as those progesterone shots had become as common place for us in the past few weeks as brushing our teeth!

I did, however, mention the growing discomfort to the nurse when she came into my room to listen to Peanut's heart rate at about 6:00 p.m. After finding a strong and reassuring heart rate, she returned to my room with an antacid. Half an hour later, with the discomfort still there and Jason getting restless, Mark decided to take him home, hoping that I would be able to get some relief from this now nagging pain after they left.

Just before they left, my mother called from Ohio and I was surprised that she could tell I was in pain even over the telephone. Her comment made me realize that the pain was increasing. Even so, I wasn't alarmed or even suspicious about the pain because, unlike uterine contractions, it was constant. And the absence of bleeding was somewhat reassuring. So, given my predisposition to having this kind of discomfort in the past, I assumed the pain would go away eventually.

Sometime around 8:00 p.m., the pain began to increase and decrease in waves. After about 45 minutes of this, I realized, as if against my own will, that I was at the end of my bed curled up on all fours. That's when it hit me, *"I'm in labor!"* At this point the obstetrical nurse in me kicked in and I paged the resident on-call to my room, something that patients just don't do! When she returned the call, I informed her I was in labor and needed her in my room immediately. I then called the Labor and Delivery unit and when one of my co-workers, Rosemarie, answered the telephone I began spewing out orders for IVs, medications, blood work, anything and everything that came to mind, as if I actually had some authority! With a head calmer than mine, she told me that she would come right to my room and see what was needed.

Right after I hung up the telephone my bag of water broke with a huge gush of fluid, and at that moment all time stopped.

All the pain stopped.

All the frenzy stopped.

I was frozen.

The fight for Peanut was over. My heart couldn't believe what my mind couldn't deny.

The resident and Rosemarie ran into the room almost at the same time and I quietly told them what happened. I laid back in the bed while the resident examined me. "The baby is in your vagina, Kathi, can you give me a push?"

"Can I give you a push?" I thought. "Are you crazy? You want me to push my baby away from me? You want *me* to finish this horrible nightmare? I can't! I won't!" Then I heard a voice in my heart. The voice said to me, "Kathi, you're the only one who can."

"But that's not fair!" I thought. "I'm his mother!" Yet I knew it was true. No one else could do this, and I knew I would hate this moment for the rest of my life. In my heart I said, "Good-bye, Peanut, my love," and with one tiny push I let my baby go.

"Rosemarie, can you tell what it is?" I asked. At this young age it can be difficult to tell. "It's a boy, Kathi," was all she said. Whispering, I replied, "My precious baby boy."

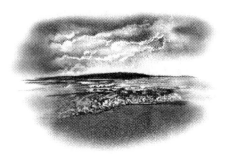

Oh, that my grief were fully weighed,
And my calamity laid with it on the scales!
For then it would be heavier
than the sand of the sea.

Job 6: 2–3

TWO

What do we do now?

OUR BABY IS gone, along with our hopes and dreams for him. So, what's next? Do we just go on living? How do we do that? For that matter, where do we find the will to do that? Look at me, physically, I look pregnant but…

These were some of the questions we faced the morning after Peanut died. Some of them were conscious, but some we wouldn't even allow ourselves to think. Even worse, there were questions we didn't ask because we did not know we should. The answers to those questions were the most difficult to accept.

I had my baby early – long before my due date, and I was struggling with the issue of not being pregnant. As I went home from the hospital and for months afterward I was keenly aware of the fact that *I should be pregnant.* I kept telling myself that once I got to my due date I would feel better. After all, at that point it would "okay" to not be pregnant. But these little pep talks to myself really didn't convince me that it was true, and I had no one to ask.

As I walked around the community, shopping, going to movies, going to church and even working in the garden, when I saw a pregnant woman I would think, "I'll bet she's due about the same time I was due. I guess that's how 'big' I would be now." The anger and pain would come again, and again I would try to remind myself of the number of weeks left until my due date, when I thought I'd feel better. With a sigh of resignation I would try to put it out of my mind.

Finally January 15th arrived. I woke up that morning and felt as though a *huge* burden had been lifted from my shoulders! This day was to be my due day and now it *really* was okay to not be pregnant! It was then I realized that I had to give myself permission to not be pregnant and I couldn't do that until my due date. What a relief it was to not feel guilty because there was no baby growing inside of me! Lesson #1.

Lesson #2. Knowledge is power: you need to know that even at the beginning of the second trimester it is possible that your milk may come in. A few days after I came home from the hospital I was hit with a physical aspect of the delivery that never entered my mind: my milk came in. I was only 16 weeks pregnant; how could this be? Why didn't anyone warn me that this might happen? Wait a minute, I'm an obstetrical nurse, why didn't I know? But then, how would I know? I took care of patients having babies. I didn't see those patients after they went home. Once again, I had no one to tell me what to expect. Doctors just don't talk about those things.

So, here I was with milk in my breasts and no baby to take it. Shocked, I felt like the victim of a cruel joke. To this was added the torturous thought that I should have known. Every mother who loses a baby this young should know to expect this!

Up until a few years ago doctors were prescribing one of two medications to help dry up breast milk for women who didn't wish to breastfeed. For the most part that practice has been discontinued, in part because these medications tend to cause the blood pressure to rise, therefore eliminating a large number of women who could receive it. In addition, studies have shown that the medicines didn't actually dry up the milk but merely delayed lactation until the medicine was stopped.

While stopping the production of milk with medications is not an option, there are things you can do to slow and eventually stop the process. You should wear a good, supportive bra 24 hours a day and decrease stimulation to your breasts as much as possible for a couple of weeks after delivering. For instance, don't let the water hit your breasts when you're in the shower. Decreasing your fluid intake slightly might also help, but be careful that you don't become dehydrated, especially in the summer. You can also take a pain reliever to ease the discomfort and achiness that often accompanies having your milk come in.

But what about the emotional pain? I found that talking to my husband and my best friend helped. They were comfortable being with me while my tears flowed. I urge you not to keep it in. Grief and burdens this heavy are a little lighter when their weight is shared with one or two others. I would also encourage you to share this burden with your God. He cares for you and wants to lessen your pain, and He's the only one who is there with you during those times when there's no one else around and you feel so very alone.

Lesson #3. Try to fight the temptation to take responsibility for the loss of your baby. During those times when you're alone, it's not unusual to play over and over in your mind the events which led up to the delivery of your baby: the pain of realizing your baby was not going to live, the difficult decisions that had to be made and perhaps feelings of guilt over what happened. It is very normal to analyze your pregnancy and how you cared for yourself and, your baby during that time. Unfortunately, this type of close examination frequently leads to feelings of guilt.

"If only I had done this, or maybe if I hadn't done that…"

Over the years many patients have expressed these feelings to me, even before they left the hospital. I also struggled long and often with this enemy of peace of mind called guilt. As I mentioned earlier, one of the things that gave me hope in both of my pregnancies during those horrendous episodes of bleeding was that I didn't have any pain. Yet, when the pain came, I didn't recognize it as a sign of labor. I mistook the signs, missed the obvious. How can that be? I work in Labor and Delivery! I've taught classes on how to recognize labor when it starts! If only I had seen it for what it was immediately, maybe we could have stopped it. I've often wondered if I am responsible for my own baby's death!

I found no peace in knowing that I had done everything within my power to keep this baby alive and healthy. Even though I adhered strictly to the doctor's order for bed rest, took every shot, pill, suppository and test that was prescribed, stopped working without complaint, and did all of this with a calmness and positive attitude that can only come from relying on God, I felt responsible and guilty. This kind of self-bashing can become a ghost that constantly haunts you. It steals your joy and affects your interactions with your husband, your other children and anyone close to you. I found the worst thing about these nagging thoughts and feelings is that there is no rest or hiding from them. They can even attack you in your sleep.

In my opinion, the best advice anyone can give regarding these guilt feelings is to talk to your husband, the father of your baby. After all, he's the one who was with you while you followed all the doctor's orders. He saw the sacrifices you made, he helped and encouraged you through those trying weeks. That is what I should have done. But I felt I couldn't. Those same thoughts that convinced me I was responsible for my child's death also caused me to wonder if Mark blamed me also. Nothing could have been further from the truth. He never said or did anything to support this vicious lie, but how could I know that – I didn't talk to him! The only thing harder than learning from experience is not learning from experience! Do yourself a favor and talk to your partner about your feelings. If the baby's father is not a part of your life, talk to the person closest to you, the one who was there beside you as you took the journey through this pregnancy and loss.

Although I let my foolish fears rule my actions and I neglected to go to Mark, I did go to the one other friend that I knew would listen, offer comfort, and give words of wisdom. I took my guilty feelings to God. It is so comforting to be able to go to Him, the One Being who has perfect control, when we are completely out of control. When you get through all of the garbage that obscures the truth, control is really what it's all about. Barbara Johnson, a woman who lost two sons at a young age and the author of *Splashes of Joy in the Cesspools of Life,* writes, "…when there is no control, there is no responsibility." This is the wisdom that God gave me slowly, over a period of time. He showed me that He wanted Peanut with Him. I didn't know why at the time and will probably never know all the reasons why during this lifetime, but I do know that He wanted Peanut with Him. Had I recognized the pain as a sign of labor and the doctors and nurses were able to stop it, they would only have prolonged the inevitable and our anguish. I now know that it was God in His goodness and mercy who allowed me to miss the "obvious" so that my suffering would be shortened. In Chapter 6 I will talk some more about how to "go to God" and how to deal with some of the other feelings resulting from the loss of a loved one, including anger.

In short, the answer to the question, "What do we do now?" is: take everything slowly. Your body is going through all the changes that every woman experiences after giving birth. Those changes happen slowly, for the most part, over a period of about six weeks.

Before you leave the hospital, you should receive written instructions regarding how the healing is expected to progress and the levels of activity that are realistic. However, if this is overlooked or if questions arise after you've left, don't hesitate to call your doctor. There are so many emotional issues to be worked out, help yourself by allowing your physician to handle the physical ones.

Let your slowly changing body be a reminder to you that your heart and your mind need time to heal also. Insisting that things return to "normal" *right now* will do nothing to speed up the process and may frustrate and discourage you even more. Allow those who love you to take care of and comfort you. You'll both feel better for it.

Whether physical or emotional, healing is not an event; it is a process. Eleven years after losing Peanut I've found that retelling our story through this book is both painful and comforting at the same time. You may find, as I did, that you will always have an empty place in your heart where your baby was. I'm always telling my patients that I have a "Peanut-sized" hole in my heart. My heart has been filled with many other people and things, but only Peanut can fill his place. While the loss of any loved one is an incredibly difficult burden to bear, I think that it is just a little more difficult to lose a baby because we don't have those precious memories and anecdotes to hold on to.

Once, I asked Mark when the hurting would stop and he wisely told me, "Never." He knew that while there *is* an end to the crushing, all-consuming pain , the longing for our baby will always be there, deep inside. Years later, you may find yourself unexpectedly facing that old pain and yearning for your baby. But, take heart: with time God and your loved ones will once again be a source of joy and laughter. In Jeremiah 31:13, God promised those who turn to Him, "I will turn their mourning to joy; I will comfort them and make them rejoice rather than sorrow."

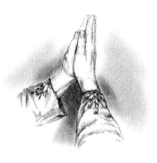

But you, O God, do see trouble and grief;
you consider it to take it in hand.

Psalm 10:14 (NIV)

THREE

Dad, there's a lot you can do to help

WHEN IT COMES to being helpful and supportive during a pregnancy, even a troubled or high-risk pregnancy, the things that the father-to-be can do to make the pregnancy a little smoother and easier are often obvious. Clothes need to be cleaned, food needs to be bought, put away and cooked, the house needs to be cleaned, and errands need to be run. Preparing the house and the baby's room for its eventual arrival is another task waiting for dad. Then there's the need for a listening ear so that fears, concerns and the complaints that result from the discomforts of pregnancy can be addressed. Oh, and don't forget going to work to support this growing family and lend some sense of "normalcy" to the household. Most dads do these things to some degree. Some chores are done cheerfully, others with more procrastination than joy! The point is, you have your work cut out for you.

If your baby dies, however, every thing can become cloudy, including the "obvious" and you may feel as though you are powerless to do anything. This is a time typically filled with shock and a sense of chaos. Often neither parent knows how to console or find comfort for themselves, let alone help their partner. This was also true for Mark and me. I am blessed to have a very sensitive husband who relies on our loving God. He's shared with me that there were times when he just didn't know what to do. During those times it was his desire to help me and his faith that "showed" him what was needed. Often, that meant just quietly staying beside me, silently praying.

Of course, the thing he struggled with the most was not being there when Peanut was born. It happened so suddenly I could only call him after the fact. When he did arrive at the hospital shortly afterward, he did the very thing I needed the most: he held me and said nothing except, "I love you." He knew that there was nothing else that could or even should be said at that moment. This was one of those moments when comfort can only be found in the arms of someone who loves you. Mark stayed with me until I fell asleep, and then quietly went home with the weight of both of our worlds on his shoulders.

The next morning we faced the cruel reality that, in spite of our loss and pain, life was going on. I would have been happy to let it go on without me. I was much too overwhelmed to be a part of it. I was in the hospital, secluded from the world, but Mark was out there and it became clear to him very quickly that there were people and things that just could not be ignored.

On the day I was discharged from the hospital, Mark arrived to take me home and was greeted by a woman who was all dressed and ready to go, including sunglasses! You see I just couldn't stop crying no matter what I did, and I didn't want the people around me to see the red eyes and the tears. So, I thought, if I covered my eyes with my sunglasses it would be as if the tears were never there! Mark knew that the tears *had* to be there and that our loved ones and friends expected them. He gently helped me realize this and slowly, patiently supported me through the first agonizing step I had to take in "going on with my life" – walking out the hospital door without my baby.

Throughout that first day home there were many people that needed to be contacted and told our sad news. Mark followed my cues regarding this chore. There were some people with whom I really wanted to speak myself, and Mark encouraged me to do that *when I was ready*. On the other hand, there were only so many times I could bring myself to say the words. When I reached that point, and it came very quickly, he stepped in and said, "Honey, tell me who you want to call and I will call them." It was a tremendous help to know that I didn't have to tackle this responsibility on my own.

Another unexpected burden that came with the loss of our child was that some very well-meaning friends began to speak of my "miscarriage." At the time, I was not at all interested in medical terms or definitions. How could anyone think of my Peanut as a "miscarriage?" How dare they trivialize his life with such a sterile word? I *did not* have a miscarriage, *I had a baby*, and my baby died. Mark not only understood how I felt, he agreed and lovingly took up the task of tactfully expressing our feelings to those who didn't understand. I was so filled with hurt and anger that, had I tried to explain how we felt, I'm sure I would have alienated some people who were only trying to help and who were struggling with this themselves.

Perhaps the question friends most frequently ask after a loss is, "Is there anything I can do?" There are often specific, practical needs, at least for a short period of time, for help with things like meals, laundry, and house cleaning. Losing a lot of blood (as I did), a cesarean delivery, enduring a long period of time in the hospital on bed rest, receiving the various drugs, and other physical ordeals can leave a woman feeling weak. Add any one of these to the overwhelming sense of loss and grief, and suddenly facing life's daily chores seems unbearable.

Mark was ready to step in, not only to cook meals but also to make arrangements with those who were willing to provide meals when he could not. When Dad makes these arrangements for Mom it really allows her to focus on working through the physical and emotional pain. This can be especially helpful if there are other little mouths to feed.

When friends asked us, "Is there anything I can do?" however, we weren't always sure what we needed. For reasons I will discuss in Chapter Five we did not have a funeral for Peanut. Perhaps the lack of a funeral, coupled with the ways that people tend to gloss over miscarriages, led most of our acquaintances to feel that it was either not necessary or just too uncomfortable to express their sympathy in any way beyond communicating it on the telephone when they first heard the news. Only one very dear person, the nurse I taught childbirth classes for, expressed her sympathy by sending us a flower arrangement. Attached was a card that read, "In memory of the joy of Peanut." When I received those flowers my tears flowed like a river. I continue to be inexpressibly grateful that at least one other person recognized the reality of Peanut's life and the joy it brought us for a short time. I still cherish that card.

We had no way of knowing that our friends and family would be so hesitant to express the sympathy we know they were feeling. Along with mentioning meals or maybe errands that need to be done, let me suggest to Dad that the caller might appreciate hearing that a card, phone call or flower arrangement would mean a lot at this time. These gestures can truly make a difference. I can confirm from my personal experience the words of Proverbs 12: 25: "Anxiety in the heart of man causes depression, but a good word makes it glad."

We often find ourselves surrounded by friends and family immediately following the loss of a loved one, only to discover that we're going it alone a month later. As you share your needs with well-wishers, encouraging them to call, visit, provide a meal, or even to send flowers a month or so from now may provide timely comfort and encouragement. Right now it's difficult to look past today, but you both will benefit if you suggest that others do.

Due to the time I was away from work during my pregnancy with Peanut I found myself in a situation where I needed to return to work two weeks after I delivered or I risked losing my position in Labor and Delivery, though I was assured of having a job somewhere in the medical center. This was just unacceptable to me. Not only did I love my job in Obstetrics, but that was where I felt I had been called by God. Of course, two weeks was too soon. I dreaded going to work and watching happy couples deliver healthy, full term babies and take those adorable children home. But I knew if I was going to stay where God wanted me I had no choice. So, two weeks after Peanut's birth and death I was back at work.

Returning to work uncovered yet another unexpected and unwanted surprise. Because I didn't recognize that I was in labor until minutes before Peanut was born and there was no time to transfer to Labor and Delivery, I delivered him in my room on the Maternity floor. It never occurred to Mark or me that my co-workers would not be informed of the delivery. Sure enough, within five minutes of being back on the unit three people said to me in one way or another that they were glad to see me back and glad that everything was okay with the baby. I managed to explain the situation calmly to the first two, but unfortunately for the third well-wisher, I broke down and had to excuse myself. How could they not know? How many times was I going to have to say that my baby was dead? Was I really strong enough to continue to work here with all the reminders that, while other babies lived and thrived, mine was gone?

While that first day back at work was one of the toughest shifts I've ever worked, my colleagues were wonderfully supportive. Once they realized what had happened, they became instrumental in making that first day a little less burdensome. However, if we had not assumed that the staff I work with were aware of our loss, Mark would have called the unit to request that a notice be posted to let them know. Dads, even if it's Mom who calls her work with the news, you might consider calling again to ask that the news be posted in the lunchroom, bulletin board or other prominent place. A little damage control can go a long way in making Mom's first day back to work a little less stressful. This might also be a consideration with church, your other children's day care center, schools or any place the family goes often.

While the question of when to return was out of our hands if I was to return to Labor and Delivery, I did wrestle with whether I could return to my old department at all. What I needed from Mark was, first to hear the pros and cons as he saw them and, secondly, to know that he would support me no matter what I decided. It's only fair to tell you, though, that what I told him I needed was for him to decide. In my heart I knew that he couldn't make that decision for me, that it was between God and myself. Fortunately, he knew that also and tenderly reminded me of it. My advice to Dads: firmly and clearly state the facts as you see them. You might be able to point out advantages and disadvantages that

Mom can't see at the moment. Firmly and lovingly assure her that you are behind her in whatever decision she makes, then firmly but gently nudge her toward making that decision as she shows signs of being ready. If all of this seems overwhelming to you, I encourage *you* to talk to someone. Don't go it alone!

In my case, I knew in my heart that God had called me to Labor and Delivery years ago and had not rescinded that call. Mark was aware that we both knew that. I am grateful that he was willing to stand by and pray for me as he gave me the time and space I needed to come to that realization on my own.

If going back to work is not an issue for your wife, you may need to go through a similar process regarding her return to church, college, places she volunteers, going home to visit family or even returning to an exercise group. You may find that she's struggling with an issue that seems trivial to you. No matter how insignificant the situation may appear to you, if she's wrestling with it, she needs your help. The relatively sudden and drastic hormonal changes Mom is experiencing can influence her perception of things. Issues she might normally view as minor can become huge obstacles. It was very comforting for me to be able to rely on someone I knew was not being affected by those physical factors and, therefore, had a somewhat better perspective.

There is one other extremely difficult issue that needs to be addressed: whether or not to try to have another baby and, if so, when. I vividly remember a well-intentioned person saying to me, "It's just too soon to think about that now. You need time to heal first." After that, every time I found myself thinking about this question I would stop and chastise myself for trying to tackle it too soon. Besides, I wondered if thinking about this so soon meant the possibility of another baby was more important to me than Peanut. But the thoughts would not go away. Looking back, I realize that when these thoughts first came to me, I wasn't yet ready to make any decisions. In part, I wasn't prepared for this because I *did* need time to focus on my Peanut and his loss. My friend was right to a certain extent. But I *did* need to talk about it. In fact, what I really needed was to be reassured that Mark was willing to discuss the possibilities when the time was right and to know that he understood that I was willing to keep our options open. In short, I just wanted to talk.

There were some things we had to do before we could make that decision. First, we had to try to gain some understanding of why this happened. In our case, we knew it was a matter of how my body responded to pregnancy and not because of a problem with Peanut. This meant that I would have to undergo various tests to determine if I was even capable of carrying another pregnancy to term. This can be a consideration if the mother has any number of chronic illnesses, including diabetes, hypertension and Lupus just to name a few. In other cases, the reason for the loss may be more apparent, such as a tight umbilical cord around the baby's neck or a knot in the umbilical cord. If this had been the situation, our concern would not have been about my ability to carry another pregnancy but rather, the chances that this kind of "cord accident" could happen again. Our doctor could have given us those statistics. A third possible reason for the loss could have been a genetic anomaly with the baby. Again further tests on the baby and possibly an autopsy might assist in making further decisions.

Whatever the cause or possible causes for the death of your precious baby, the time to talk about other children is *when you are ready*. Dad can definitely help in this area by letting Mom know that he is willing to discuss this with her whenever she is ready. This kind of flexibility is asking a lot– what do you do if she's ready to talk about it and you're not? The possibility of that happening is one of the things that makes this issue so difficult. My suggestion to Dad is twofold. First and foremost, share your thoughts and feelings with someone close to you that you trust preferably another man. Perhaps you could go to your clergy, father, brother or best friend. Seek guidance and perspective from any one of these people, so that you do not feel as though you are facing this weighty challenge on your own. The mother of your baby is getting strength and courage from you; please don't be afraid to look for the same for yourself from others who care about you.

My second piece of advice is that the two of you do as much as you can to get all of your questions answered. In addition to some of the questions mentioned above, you may also have financial questions, especially if you are suffering from infertility, which can put a tremendous strain on a family's budget. All of these considerations need to be dealt with before you can even begin to take on the toughest question of this issue: Are we emotionally prepared and capable of facing the challenges of another pregnancy? This question not only requires introspection and discussion between the two of you, but also much prayer, individually and together as a couple. The Bible tells us in Ecclesiastes 4:12, "Though one may be overpowered by another, two can withstand him. And a threefold cord is not quickly broken." Should you decide to have another baby, that "cord of three strands" will help to make those nine months much more smooth.

It is only after (1) your doctor has answered your questions regarding the physical aspects of this decision, (2) you've faced the realities of the influence of your personal finances in regard to another pregnancy, and (3) you've searched yourselves and God, that you can come to the place where you can feel confident in reaching informed, realistic conclusions regarding the emotional stress of trying all over again.

Dads, I've handed you a plate-full, or should I say life has handed you a plate-full. In the next two chapters I'll address a few additional things that the two of you may need to walk through together. The truth of the matter is that there are very few things in relationship to the loss of your baby and "moving on" in life that either of you should attempt to tackle on your own. I urge you to draw strength from each other as you contin-ue this part of your life's journey.

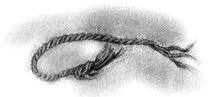

Two are better than one,
Because they have a good reward for their labor.
For if they fall, one will lift up his companion.
But woe to him who is alone when he falls,
For he has no one to help him up.
Again, if two lie down together,
they will keep warm;
But how can one be warm alone?
Though one may be overpowered by another,
two can withstand him.
And a threefold cord is not quickly broken.

Ecclesiastes 4: 9-12

FOUR

What do we tell the kids?

MY FIRST THOUGHT after calling Mark to tell him that Peanut was gone was of Jason. How do I tell that precious child who has been anticipating the arrival of his brother or sister for three months that he will never get to see Peanut? How do I say, in the same sentence, that he had a brother and his brother was dead? Several different approaches came to mind. The first one was that we just wouldn't tell him and he would forget about it. Did I mention that grief mixed with rapidly changing hormones can really influence a woman's thinking?! For just a fleeting moment I *really* did think that this was a possible alternative. Of course, I knew we had to tell him.

Next, I thought: okay, if we have to tell him then maybe we didn't have to tell him. Maybe

Mark could tell him while I took a vacation in the Bahamas! No, there were a lot of things Mark could do for me in the next few days and weeks, but it wouldn't be fair to Mark or Jason if we didn't do this together. Unfortunately, those were the only two ideas I liked! Any other alternative involved me actually looking Jason in the eyes and telling him.

So, until Mark arrived to take me home I filled my time coming up with scripts. It's absolutely amazing how many ways a person can say the exact same thing! But, it was devastating to know that at the end of each script was Jason's five-year-old heart being broken. As you can imagine, I was filled with turmoil every waking moment until Mark arrived.

As soon as Mark walked into the room, I hit him with it. "When should we tell Jason? What should we tell Jason? Where should we tell Jason? Who should start? What are you going to say? What am I going to say? Could we tell him next February?" Mark patiently waited until the barrage of questions subsided, asked me if I was finished and quietly said that he thought we should tell Jason as soon as we got home so that it wouldn't be hanging over us. He said he would get me settled in bed in our room and we would tell him. We would tell him that the baby in my belly was a boy and that the baby went to Heaven.

As you can see, it was a good thing that I had

come up with all of my elaborate scenarios because Mark was a wreck!

I knew in my heart that he was right. The best thing was to tell Jason immediately. We certainly didn't want him to hear this news accidentally from someone else. We needed to tell him as truthfully and as simply as we could. Even stated in the simplest way possible, it would be a horrible piece of information for his five-year-old mind to process, especially considering the fact that my 31-year-old mind was not doing a very good job sifting through this!

With dread, hesitation and my sunglasses I went home from the hospital. After a very enthusiastic greeting from my incredibly special Jason (our children can be so good for our egos!) and the removal of my sunglasses after several of "those looks" from Mark, I went upstairs while Jason and Mark prepared something for each of us to drink. They made themselves comfortable and we talked for a few minutes about how nice it was for us to all be back together again.

Then Mark began, "Jason, the baby that was in Mommy's belly, Peanut, it was a baby boy."

Jason's eyes lit up the room, "A boy!"

"Yes, sweetheart. But Peanut went up to heaven to be with God."

The sparkle, instantly gone, was replaced by a questioning look, a look that said, "Daddy and Mommy can fix anything. Fix this." We sat in silence for what seemed like hours. Then Jason threw himself facedown onto the bed and, pounding his fists repeatedly into the mattress, screamed, "My brother is dead! My brother is dead! My brother is dead!" As Mark and I hugged each other and sobbed, I was surprised that Jason was so instantly attached to Peanut as his brother. I knew our baby was a boy and, therefore, our son and Jason's brother. I just didn't realize that Jason would grasp that so quickly and feel such a bond to Peanut because of that relationship. How short-sighted of me.

After about thirty seconds of fist pounding, we all hugged and cried together. Slowly, the tears subsided and we just hugged. Finally, Mark said that he thought I should get some rest. Right before they left the room, Mark told Jason that after a woman has a baby there are chemicals (hormones) in her body that can cause her to cry for no apparent reason. He told Jason that if that happened he should quietly hug me and know that there was nothing seriously wrong. I can't express how much that meant to me. First, Mark was communicating to Jason that we did, indeed, have a baby. Secondly, he was attempting to put Jason at ease if he saw Mommy crying and didn't know why. What a wonderfully loving thing for him to say for the benefit of both of us.

Jason went to his room, Mark went down to the living room, and I lay down in a feeble attempt to take a nap. Although I was physically

and emotionally exhausted, my mind was spin-
ning with all that had taken place in one short
yet extremely long week, so I ended up just lying
there – thinking. It wasn't long after Jason left
the room that he timidly walked back in again.
"Mommy, I think I know what will cheer you
up", he said.

"You do? And what would that be, my
love?"

"I think we should play 'Thunder Cats!'"

Smiling, I said, "You know, I think you're
right!" It occurred to me that Jason had reacted
to our terrible news both as badly as I feared
he would and as well as I hoped and prayed he
would. I marvel at the resilience of children and
continue to be blessed by their ability to give
us "grown-ups" a more mature perspective on
things for which there is really no understanding.

As we played together, slowly he began to
ask questions about his brother. What did he
look like? Did Peanut look like Jason? How big
was he? And so on. It was a very special time
for us, and it set the stage for future questions
and discussions about this person who remains
so very dear to us.

A few days later, I was sitting on the edge on
our bed with my back to the door, putting some
clothes away, when Jason walked into the room.
He walked around to the side of the bed I was
sitting on, sat down beside me, put his little hand

on my knee and said, "Mommy, is this one of those times? Would you like a hug?" His tenderness and understanding touched my heart and I smiled at him and said, "No, sweetheart, this is not one of those times, but I could use a hug from you anytime!" Our children understand so much – sometimes even more than we.

Almost every day for quite a while after that someone in the family, and often it was Jason, spoke of Peanut. To this day, many years later, his name still comes up in family discussion, in the way that you would speak of any other family member that was gone. "I wonder what Peanut would look like now." "How would he like this person or that person?" "He would be _____ years old now." Peanut was born into our family, and the three of us know that he will always be a part of it.

Now that you know how we handled this situation and the outcome, how does that apply to you? To be honest, I just don't know. But I would encourage you to be honest with your children--not an honesty is that filled with details, but a simple honesty. Listen very carefully to their questions and try not to give them more information than their questions are asking. While there is little you can do to make their pain go away beyond being there to love and support them, you can ease the natural apprehension you have regarding breaking the news to them by reminding yourself that children, especially those with support from their families, have an ability to "rise above" and go on. If you watch them and listen, really listen, they often teach us, through example, how to handle tough situations more gracefully. Above all, allow them the freedom to talk about and ask questions regarding their baby brother or sister. Making the baby "go away" in family discussions won't erase the memory of the baby in their minds and will only leave a lot of questions unanswered.

Again, I would also suggest that you rely on our loving, tender God to help get your family through this. When we face situations that are completely beyond our control, we do well to turn those times over to God. Psalm 55:22 reassures us that God is faithful to His children: "Cast your burden on the LORD, and He shall sustain you." He is truly a wonderful God and is in control even when we're not!

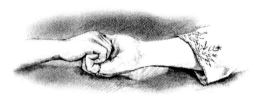

"… and a little child will lead them."

Isaiah 11:6

FIVE

You can celebrate your child

As I MENTIONED earlier, one of the main purposes of this book is to help other couples through the devastating wilderness we find ourselves in after the loss of a baby. Some of the things I've shared were the result of the good decisions we made as we struggled through this season of our lives. Unfortunately, one thing I would have done differently is that I would have celebrated Peanut more openly.

Because I had worked in a Labor and Delivery unit for eight years before Peanut was born, I had learned a lot about the value of not only acknowledging the baby that was lost but celebrating him or her. I had learned the importance of this celebration and believed then, as I still do today, that it is important for Mom and Dad to not only see their baby after it is born but also hold him or her. Having said that, you might be surprised to learn that when Rosemarie asked me if I wanted to see the baby on the awful night he was born, without hesitation I said, "No."

Grief can have a very real effect on how we think, or don't think, things through. At that moment I was actually thinking like a nurse. I had been present at the premature delivery of far too many four- to five-month-old babies, and all I could think was that there isn't much that distinguishes one baby from another, at least physically, at this point in development. They all have little to no hair, their eyes aren't open to be able to determine the color, and it's hard to even see if there are any dimples.

"But this baby is different," I thought. "This baby is *my* baby!" Subconsciously, I was afraid that I would not be able to find anything different about Peanut. The thing that my grief was disguising was that it really didn't matter whether or not I could find anything physically different about our Peanut. I was right, he *was* in fact different; it didn't matter if he looked like thousands of other babies or like no baby ever born. He was different because he was mine. That should have given me the freedom to just hold my baby boy, but my fear won over, and I never saw my Peanut.

Now, I know that I will indeed see and hold Peanut someday in heaven, and with time I became content with that knowledge. Unfortunately, my decision to not see him affected someone else. As Jason and I sat on my bed the day I came home from the hospital, and played and talked about Peanut, I found myself in the uncomfortable position of having to tell him that I never saw his brother. Jason was not happy with me, to say the least! How could I not look at him? How would he ever know what his brother looked like? I felt both uncomfortable and apologetic as I tried to explain myself to this little boy.

Of course, I cannot change the past but, if it's not too late, I strongly advise you to hold your baby. I had always encouraged my patients to see and hold their babies, but now I have a greater appreciation of how special that can be. I have not once had a mom or dad tell me that they wish they hadn't seen the baby.

Your nurse will probably offer to do several other things for you after the delivery that will help keep the baby's memory alive for you. Things like taking pictures of the baby, especially in clothing that the hospital will provide and that you can keep; taking footprints of the baby; giving you the tape measure that was used to measure the baby's length; keeping an identification bracelet with the information of the baby's delivery; and cutting off a lock of the baby's hair for you to keep. Some hospitals will even offer you a certificate of life with the baby's name and birth date on it. The hospital I work at provides very pretty decorated boxes in which you can keep the mementos. If your hospital doesn't offer this, it might be a nice family project to get materials from a local craft store and make your own box.

Naming the baby is also something I would highly encourage. Mark and I discussed giving Peanut another, more traditional name and we decided that no matter what we named the baby no name would be as natural as Peanut. We did, however, speak with Jason's kindergarten teacher about what had happened and told him that Jason was very proud of his little brother, Peanut. We were concerned that some of his classmates might not understand Peanut's unusual name and laugh. The important thing is not so much what the baby's name is, but that he or she has one.

Finally there is the issue of whether to have a funeral for the baby. Again, I would encourage you to have some form of gathering to celebrate the baby's life. Funeral homes are experienced in providing this service for parents and can help guide you through your decisions in this area. Peanut's body was cremated and there was a small service at the cemetery where the ashes were buried. As with the decision to name the baby, it really isn't a matter of what you do but rather that you do something. Having friends and family gather around you to express their love and support can really help to make this incredibly difficult time just a little easier. We were not created to be islands; isolation only makes the grief more painful.

There are so many other things you can do to express your love for, and memory of, this special person in your lives. Planting a special tree, making a donation to a charity – especially those that benefit children, writing a poem or story about the baby, designing and having a special piece of jewelry with the baby's birthstone and/or name in it, making a shadow box with the mementos you have from the hospital, are just a few of the ways you can memorialize your special baby. As with most things, the only ones who can decide what is best for your family are the two of you. If we choose to welcome our live newborns into our families in the various ways that fit us, then certainly we should exercise the same freedom to memorialize our babies in our own special way.

POSSIBLE MEMENTOS FOR YOUR BABY'S MEMORY BOX

A locket of hair
The baby's blanket
A few dried flowers
Pictures of the baby
Mass or prayer cards
A copy of the baby's footprints
The program from the baby's funeral
This book with the journal completed
The gown the baby wore in the pictures
The measuring tape used at the hospital
One of the baby's identification bracelets
A poem, possibly written by a family member
Cards, including those that accompany flowers
A short note written by each family member to
the baby
A small stuff animal or rattle used in the baby's
pictures

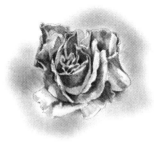

To everything there is a season,
A time for every purpose under heaven:
A time to be born, And a time to die;
A time to plant, And a time
to pluck what is planted;
A time to kill, And a time to heal;
A time to break down, And a time to build up;
A time to weep, And a time to laugh;
A time to mourn, And a time to dance;
A time to cast away stones,
And a time to gather stones;
A time to embrace, And a time
to refrain from embracing;
A time to gain, And a time to lose;
A time to keep, And a time to throw away;
A time to tear, And a time to sew;
A time to keep silence, And a time to speak;
A time to love, And a time to hate;
A time of war, And a time of peace.

Ecclesiastes 3: 1-8

SIX

Where does strength come from?

I HAVE WRITTEN QUITE a bit about the support and strength we get from our spouses, children, families, friends, and co-workers. While I do not want to minimize that in any way, there is no avoiding the reality that there are times, especially at night, when it's just me. Where does my strength come from when everyone is gone and it's just me? I can still remember times when I was alone and I thought I would go mad with grief. I would wonder if there was something wrong with me.

This is probably the most difficult time in the grieving process. Everyone has been so kind, generous, loving, and supportive and while it does help, it's just not enough. In order to gain some understanding of what is happening and how to deal with it, I'd like to take a look at the grieving process itself.

I have long appreciated the work of the late Swiss-born psychiatrist, Elisabeth Kubler-Ross. In her groundbreaking book, *On Death and Dying*, she identifies five psychological stages of grieving: denial and isolation, anger, bargaining, depression and, finally, acceptance. She is careful to say that we do not go through these stages in any particular order and, in fact, we can return to any of the stages. She asserts that grieving is not pathological in nature but, rather, a necessary response to help in healing from the overwhelming sense of loss when a loved one dies. I won't go into the details of each of these stages but highly recommend her book.

Understanding the stages of grief can provide comfort by confirming that what you are thinking and feeling is normal. We all go through each of these stages as we work through the loss of someone dear. There are, however, things you can do to help yourself travel the road to healing more gracefully.

NUTRITION

It is not uncommon to unconsciously change your eating habits, either by over- or under-eating. In both cases, it is important to know that these changes are normal and probably temporary. It is also important to try to make the foods that you do eat as nutritious as possible. Fruits are a good choice because they don't require preparation but are full of vitamins. And the natural sugar in fruits can help satisfy a "sweet tooth." If you've never taken supplements before, this would probably be a good time to add at least a multivitamin to your diet.

EXERCISE

You might find it difficult to motivate yourself to exercise at this time. But keep in mind that exercise can come in many different forms. Just taking a walk is more exercise than sitting in your room. Doing some spring cleaning, walking around the mall (this is especially good in bad weather), and gardening are just a few activities that can provide exercise. Of course, traditional jogging, working out, swimming, etc. are also beneficial in helping to relieve stress as well as providing some "alone" time to process thoughts and feelings.

GETTING REST

As with your diet, your may find that you are either sleeping all the time or you can't sleep well at all. If you are finding it difficult to sleep, getting some exercise could prove helpful. Especially in the first few weeks after losing your baby, you may find that you just don't want to get out of bed. If so, stay in bed a little longer. This is also temporary and right now you need the rest. Grief is both physically and emotionally draining. It is important and wise to listen to what your body is telling you.

ALLOW YOURSELF TO EXPRESS YOUR EMOTIONS

I happen to be one of those people who don't like to cry. I never got it when I would hear someone say, "I went to that movie and had a good cry." What exactly is a good cry?! But in the days and weeks after we lost Peanut, I began to notice that if I tried to suppress my tears I would often actually feel nauseated. In part, I was afraid if I started crying I might not stop. I can tell you from personal experience that there is an end to the tears, but it takes much longer to get to the end if you don't allow yourself to begin. If you're like me you might feel more comfortable with your tears if you go into your room by yourself and shut the door. No matter how or where you cry, I think you will find that you feel better after releasing all the emotion that can become bottled up inside you.

JOURNALING

The only journaling I had done prior to becoming pregnant with Peanut was to keep a prayer journal documenting the things I prayed about and how and when God answered my prayers. So, it really didn't occur to me that journaling would be something that would prove helpful or therapeutic as I began to process losing Peanut.

However, about seven years ago, my prayer journal started to become a more expository type of writing and I began to see the value of journaling. I've also learned that there really are no "rules" when it comes to journaling. As with most things that are new, getting started can be difficult. This can be especially true when grief is added to the experience. My suggestion is to sit down with a pen and pad and just write down what comes to mind. It might be helpful to write about what your grief feels like – does it have a color, sound, taste? Does it affect how you see things? Is today a good day? What is a good day for you? These are just a few questions to get you started. My guess is that once you get started, continuing won't be a problem. I have included a short journal after the Recommended Resources section of this book to give you a place to begin.

Journaling also provides a safe place to express or vent anger. It's a place you can "voice" your anger toward yourself, your spouse, God, your doctor, the obnoxious guy on TV selling cars–anyone, anything! Because it's for your eyes only, you don't have to worry about hurting someone's feelings or saying something that you will later regret or about which you will need to apologize. And I have found that God would prefer to hear my anger rather than my silence. He does ask, however, that I be willing to "listen" to Him as He "speaks" to my heart.

Going back to read through your journal a week, month, or year later will show you how much you've healed and how it happened. It may also prove quite valuable if you are in a position in the future to walk through the grieving process with a friend or co-worker.

Talking and Reading about Grief and Grieving

There are many avenues available today to help you express your thoughts and feelings, as well as to hear the thoughts and feelings of others. These resources can be quite helpful in confirming that what you're going through is normal; they can also give you some ideas about coping mechanisms that you might not otherwise have considered.

Support groups provide one such avenue. Many of these can be found on the Internet. Speaking with a trained professional – psychiatrist, psychologist, or clergy – can help. Seek out a person or group that you feel you can trust: we humans are not likely to open up regarding our feelings unless we know we can trust those who are listening and sharing with us.

Many books have been written on the subject of loss and grieving. I have included a recommended resource list at the end of this book.

Of course, this list is not all-inclusive but it may prove helpful in getting you started. Gaining knowledge from any of these sources can empower and equip you for the really tough days.

Focusing on reading may feel like an insurmountable challenge right now. Many of the books that I've suggested in Recommended Resources are available as audio books. This might be a way of hearing the thoughts, feelings, and suggestions of others who have been through this struggle without the added stress of forcing yourself to read.

In the Recommended Resources list I have included all the information I was able to find. You will find that in some cases the publisher and/or year of publication are missing. In spite of this, you will be able to find each of these resources by using any of the popular search engines on the internet.

———

As I have alluded throughout the book, I am not an expert in the area of grieving and I feel certain that you will discover even better suggestions from the sources that I've listed above. Having said that, you may have already begun to realize for yourself that there is an "expertise" that comes from being thrust into a situation that you would never have chosen for yourself; it is from that "expertise" that I have written. However, I cannot close without emphasizing the strength, especially in the middle of the night, that comes from Him who keeps you and will not slumber (Psalm 121:3).

As wonderful as Mark was in the days and weeks following Peanut's death, there still were things that I couldn't share with him, not due to any fault of his or mine; some times there are things so deep in the soul that we cannot put words to them. It was at these times that I found great strength and comfort from the knowledge that, "Likewise the Spirit also helps in our weaknesses. For we do not know what we should pray for as we ought, but the Spirit Himself makes intercession for us with groanings which cannot be uttered." (Romans 8:26) The God who created me knows me so well that He knows my greatest needs even when I can't find the words to express them to Him myself. I am so grateful that I don't have to worry about saying the right thing in the right way for God to hear me. "Father, help me," is all that is needed.

Because of what the Bible refers to as the "fellowship of suffering," if you have suffered the loss of a baby, my soul has become linked with yours in that loss. It is that bond between us that creates a longing in me for you to know the faithfulness of the God of Comfort for yourself. You will see on the recommended resources page a CD entitled, "Comfort." I strongly encourage you to get it. I believe you will find in it a sooth-ing "bath" for your soul.

Finally, over the next weeks, months and years, as you begin to find comfort and heal-ing, let me suggest that you can also make some sense out of the senseless if you take the lessons that you're learning now and share them with someone else who is suffering. That, my dear friend, will be one the greatest memorials you will ever build to the loving presence and impact that your sweet baby will always have in your life. Please know that because you have picked up this book I am praying for you.

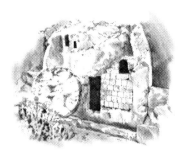

Blessed be the God and Father
of our Lord Jesus Christ,
the Father of mercies and God of all comfort,
who comforts us in all our tribulation,
that we may be able to comfort those
who are in any trouble,
with the comfort with which we
ourselves are comforted by God.

2 Corinthians 1: 3-4
(Emphasis mine)

RECOMMENDED RESOURCES

BOOKS

Beyond Grief: A Guide to Recovering From the Death of a Loved One, by C. Staudacher (1987), Human Horizon Series.

Grief's Courageous Journey: A Workbook, by S. Caplan and G. Lang (1995).

Grieving God's Way, Margaret Brownley, Winepress Publishing.

Grief...Reminders for Healing, Gale Massey, Massey Publishing, Inc.

Healing Activities for Children, Gay McWhorter, M.Ed. and ADEC Certified Grief Counselor.

Healing Grief, Amy Hillyard Jensen, Medic Publishing Company.

How to Survive the Loss of a Love: Fifty-Eight Things to Do When There Is Nothing to Be Done, by M. Colgrove, H.H. Bloomfield, and P. McWilliams (1977).

I'll Hold You in Heaven, by Jack Hayford, Regal Books (1990).

Inside Grief - Death, Loss and Bereavement - An Anthology, Line Wise, Wise Press. A thoughtful book of poetry that represents the thoughts of 37 different poets about grief.

The Kaleidoscope of Grief: When Children Experience Death. An interactive book for Children ages 7 and up.

Loss and Grief Recovery - Caring for Children with Disabilities, Chronic, or Terminal Illness, by Joyce M. Ashton with Dennis D. Ashton, Baywood Publishing Co., Inc.

Men & Grief- A Guide for Men Surviving the Death of a Loved One : A Resource for Caregivers and Mental Health Professional, by C. Staudacher (1992).

Parents' Grief - Help and Understanding After the Death of a Baby, Carol Parrott, R.N., Medic Publishing Company.

Rainbows and Rain: Finding Comfort In Times of Loss, by Peggy Waterfall, BookSurge, LLC, 2005.

Sibling Grief, Marcia G. Scherago, M.S.W., Medic Publishing Company.

Sit Down God ... I'm Angry, R.F. Smith Jr., Judson Press.

Solomon & Lily, Allie Schield and illustrated by Barb Jerome. This is a unique story about friendship, loss, transformation, healing, reaching full potential and coming full circle. The story uses the life cycle of a monarch butterfly to illustrate these themes.

What Color is Death, Daddy? An interactive book for children ages 3-7, by Joanne Cacciatore. M.I.S.S. Publishing, 2000.

When Bad Things Happen to Good People, by H.S. Kushner, Avon Books (1981).

When Someone Very Special Dies - Children Can Learn to Cope with Death , Marge Heegaard, Woodland Press. A workbook to help children deal with their feeling about death. Here is a practical format for allowing children to understand the concept of death and develop coping skills for life. Children, with adult supervision, are invited to illustrate and personalize their loss through art. This workbook encourages the child to identify support systems and personal strengths.

TAPES, CD's, DVD's

Comfort CD, Refuge records

Childhood Loss and Family Issues, Heartsounds Center DVD

Heaven's Not A Crying Place (Video Tape Version), Joey O'Connor, Revell

Where Do I Go From Here? (audio tape version), Ken Medema and Janice Winchester Nadeau, Ph.D., with Brad Walton

WEB SITES

The Comfort CD Project, www.ccphilly.org/audio/comfort.aspx

Deeper Still, www.grieving.org/

The Dougy Center for Grieving Children and Families, www.dougy.org/

Elisabeth Kubler Ross, www.elisabethkublerross.com

Healthy Grieving, www.mtch.edu/counseling/healthy_grieving.htm

Help Guide: Mental Health Issues, www.helpguide.org/mental/grief_loss.htm

Grief: God's Way of Healing the Heart (a book), www.texasstar.net/autumn/grief1.html
Grief Resources Catalog, www.griefresourcescatalog.com/catalog/

The Greiving Teen, www.americanhospice.org/articles/grievingteen.htm

YOUR BABY'S JOURNAL

_____

_____

_____

_____

_____

_____

_____

_____

_____

_____

_____

_____

_____

_____

_____

_____

_____

_____

_____

_____

_____

_____

_____

_____

_____

_____

_____

_____

_____

_____

_____

_____

_____

_____

_____

_____

_____

_____

_____

_____

_____

_____

_____

_____

_____

_____

_____

_____

_____

_____

_____

_____

_____

_____

_____

_____

_____

_____

_____

_____

_____

_____

_____

_____

_____

_____

_____

_____

_____

_____

_____

_____

_____

_____

_____

_____

_____

_____

_____

_____

_____

_____

_____

_____

_____

_____

_____

_____

_____

_____

_____

_____

_____

_____

_____

_____

_____

_____

_____

_____

_____

_____

_____

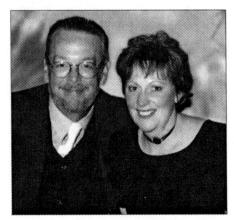

Kathi and Mark Evans

ABOUT THE AUTHOR

KATHI IS A registered nurse who has worked in Labor and Delivery for 27 years. She is certified in inpatient obstetrics and childbirth education and presently works as a staff nurse in an urban hospital in Upland, Pennsylvania that averages around 200 deliveries per month. She also participates and assists in the leadership of an average of 2 short term missions per year primarily to "third world" countries. The Evans' attend Calvary Chapel of Delaware County, Pa., where she leads the drama ministry, participates in the Arts Team, and ministers in the women's, teen, and children's ministries. She and her husband, Mark, live in Chester, Pennsylvania with their son, Jason, and her mother-in-law, Jane.

CPSIA information can be obtained at www.ICGtesting.com
Printed in the USA
LVOW11s1713210316

480094LV00001B/17/P

9 781587 367304